Table of Contents

Text Copyright © Julia Price 3

Introduction..4

What is the DASH Diet?...5

Health Benefits of the DASH Diet..7

The DASH Dietary Program 9

Why the DASH Diet Truly Works for Weight Loss and Blood Pressure 11

The Importance of Exercises 13

HEALTHY BREAKFAST 15

Omelet with chicken breast 16

Scrambled eggs with vegetables 17

Italian frittata with vegetables... 18

Pie with carrots and cheese 19

Egg rolls with vegetables 20

Cauliflower with cream cheese and chicken 21

Oatmeal with berries and muesli...22

Granola bar with cocoa and coconut 23

Cheesecake with lemon and cream cheese 24

Smoothies with chokeberry, apple, and banana 25

Smoothies with pumpkin, apple, and banana....................26

HEALTHY LUNCHES 27

Pancakes with spinach and cottage cheese 28

Zucchini Lasagna with mixed cheeses 29

Broccoli cream soup.. 30

Cream soup with chickpeas and pumpkin 31

Cream- soup with vegetables 32

Chicken baked with spinach 33

Vegetables baked in foil...34

Soup with spinach and salmon 35

Fish broth with spices 36

Baked seafood with vegetables and lemon.........................37

Baked salmon with herbs 38

Trout baked with tomatoes..39

HEALTHY SALADS & SEAFOOD 40

Salad with avocado, pineapple, and onions 41

Salad with scallops and tomatoes....................................42

Shrimp with spinach 43

Salad with mussels and pine nuts....................................44

Baked lobster with herbs...45

Chicken Breast with Persimmon 46

Chinese Pak Choy cabbage with Shrimps 47

Salad with fresh vegetables 48

Salad with shrimps, quail eggs, and black olives 49

HEALTHY DINNERS 50

Cherry dumplings... 51

Risotto with shrimps 52

Chicken breast with mushrooms......................................53

Turkey steaks 54

Vegetable stew with mushrooms 55

Fried rice with vegetables...56

Baked pork with rosemary 57

Conclusion 58

Author's Afterthoughts...59

Text Copyright © Julia Price

Legal & Disclaimer

The information contained in this book and its contents is not designed to replace or take the place of any form of medical or professional advice; and is not meant to replace the need for independent medical, financial, legal or other professional advice or services, as may be required. The content and information in this book has been provided for educational and entertainment purposes only.

The content and information contained in this book has been compiled from sources deemed reliable, and it is accurate to the best of the Author's knowledge, information and belief. However, the Author cannot guarantee its accuracy and validity and cannot be held liable for any errors and/or omissions. Further, changes are periodically made to this book as and when needed. Where appropriate and/or necessary, you must consult a professional (including but not limited to your doctor, attorney, financial advisor or such other professional advisor) before using any of the suggested remedies, techniques, or information in this book.

Upon using the contents and information contained in this book, you agree to hold harmless the Author from and against any damages, costs, and expenses, including any legal fees potentially resulting from the application of any of the information provided by this book. This disclaimer applies to any loss, damages or injury caused by the use and application, whether directly or indirectly, of any advice or information presented, whether for breach of contract, tort, negligence, personal injury, criminal intent, or under any other cause of action.

You agree to accept all risks of using the information presented inside this book.

You agree that by continuing to read this book, where appropriate and/or necessary, you shall consult a professional (including but not limited to your doctor, attorney, or financial advisor or such other advisor as needed) before using any of the suggested remedies, techniques, or information in this book.

Introduction

Probably every adult person underwent changes in blood pressure. Hypertonic disease or high blood pressure is a condition in which blood moves along the vessels to all parts of the body with tremendous force after each contraction of the heart, or rather under high pressure.

The danger of arterial hypertension is that it begins as a violation of the regulation of blood pressure, but in the future, it can lead to many serious diseases of internal organs and systems, as well as to dangerous cardiovascular diseases. Hypertensive disease, which occurs without medical supervision, can lead to heart attack, increased heart and heart failure. In the blood vessels, enlargements or aneurysms may appear which often lead to the formation of a thrombus. Because of increased blood pressure, there is a risk of cerebral hemorrhage and stroke. Hypertension can also lead to kidney failure, blindness, and various cognitive impairments, for example, memory, intelligence, and performance.

Especially dangerous are the consequences of hypertension for those who are under the influence of harmful factors such as smoking, drinking, unhealthy diet, sedentary lifestyle, frequent stress, excess weight, very high cholesterol in the body and diabetes. These people are at increased risk of heart attack, stroke and kidney failure.

In order to prevent the development of hypertension and diagnose it at the initial stage of development, you need to monitor blood pressure constantly. If you find the first symptoms of this disease, you should consult a doctor.

However, some people just need to change their way of life and get rid of bad habits, for example, to quit smoking, alcohol, as well as the rejection of salty foods and a diet that will help get rid of overweight.

As a rule, doctors recommend:

- using healthy diet, refusing fast food, and reducing the consumption of fats and salt;
- give up alcohol and smoking habits;
- increase life activity and do physical exercises at least 30 minutes a day;
- get rid of overweight and constant weight control. In fact, overweight loss promotes depression of blood pressure;
- to be positive about life and be protected from stress.

Therefore, my book is devoted to one of the methods of prevention, not only with hypertension but also with overweight. Today, I would like to tell you about a DASH diet that was originally developed for people who have a hypertensive disease, but as it turned out later, it helps ordinary people to get rid of overweight. So, let us try the DASH diet together!

Good luck!

What is the DASH Diet?

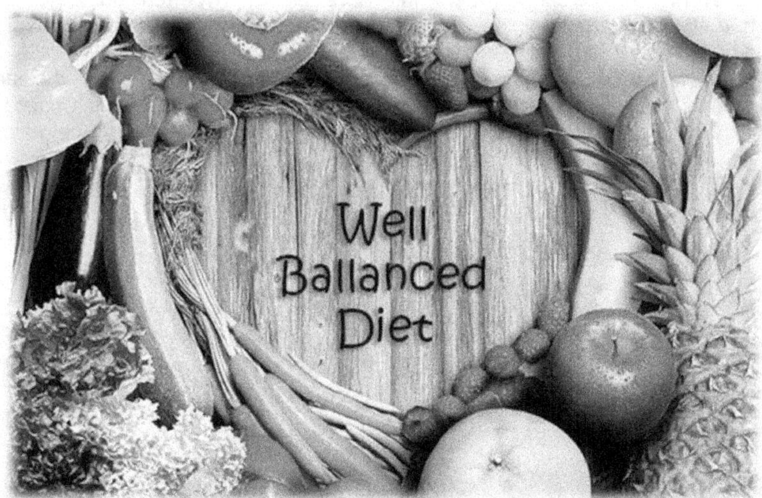

I would like to remind you that hypertension is one of the most common and frequently occurring diseases. This disease does not disappear during treatment and it is always associated with overweight problems. You can only control it and alleviate the symptoms. Many people believe that get rid of hypertension is not possible. However, today we have a hope that we will have a happy future! No, I do not have Aladdin's lamp.

Alternately, I offer you realistic way to control hypertension disease and quick method to get rid of overweight. I am talking about a popular healthy, DASH diet.

The idea of the DASH diet originated in the United States 20 years ago. Specialists and cardiologists concerned about the growing number of people suffering from high blood pressure. They decided to create a special diet to treat hypertension without pills. The result of five years of work of scientists was a new concept the DASH diet (Dietary Approaches to Stop Hypertension). As it turned out also new diet helps to lose overweight! Moreover, we already know that high blood pressure and overweight are interrelated. People, who followed the DASH diet, were able to maintain the blood pressure parameters and their weight! Thus, a therapeutic diet was in the center of attention of thousands of ordinary people who would like to improve your health and lose weight comfortably and without harm to health.

The DASH diet is a special diet regime designed to treat high blood pressure. In addition, thanks to the DASH diet, you can quickly lose weight. As you understand initially, the DASH diet was developed as a way to treat hypertension. However, studies and reviews proved the effectiveness of the diet is associated not only with improving heart function, normalizing the level of cholesterol, lowering blood pressure but also doctors summarized the significant progress in the process of losing weight and improving metabolic processes. In addition, the DASH diet can be used as a prevention of cardiovascular diseases, diabetes, kidney disease, and cancer.

For a long time, the Dash diet was considered the most popular diet among all diets, including wellness, as well as among the ways of preventing diabetes. It also occupied one of the leading positions among the regimens of nutrition for improving health effects on the heart. In the ratings for ease and convenience, as well as in the ratings on the effectiveness of weight loss, it was in the top ten.

The healthy diet includes a balanced content of the important for the normal pressure substances, such as potassium, calcium, protein, and fiber. The DASH is a balanced healthy diet that prevents and lowers high blood pressure, namely hypertension. Such a healthy approach to nutrition, in my opinion, is the key to reducing high blood pressure and diet at the same time, which effectively reduces your overweight.

This is why the DASH diet can easily reduce weight, improve health and cleanse the body of toxins. However, when using a diet, most people must take into account the metabolic, genetic characteristics of their body. Do not forget that before starting a diet, you need to check the condition of all organs and body systems. Otherwise, the harm of a diet can be irreparable. Take care and be healthy!

Good luck!

Health Benefits of the DASH Diet

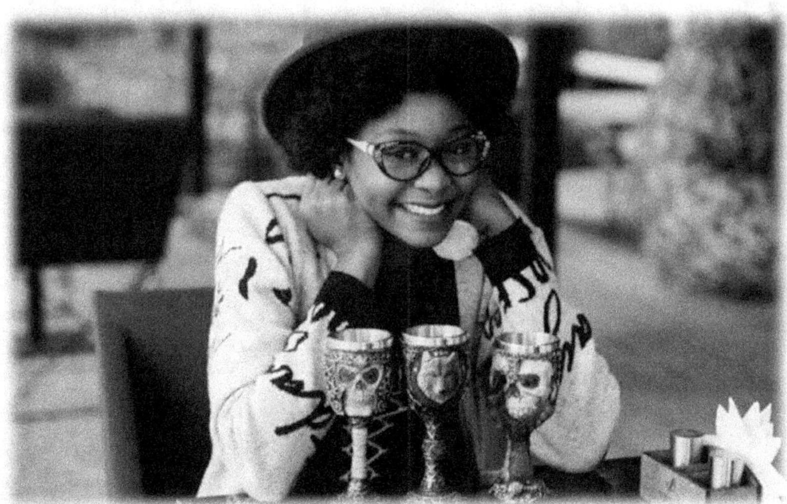

The overweight problems frequently lead to serious health consequences such as cardiovascular diseases, mainly heart disease and stroke, and diabetes, muscular-skeletal injuries, such as osteoarthritis, and some cancers, for instance, cancer of the endometrium, breast death, and colorectal carcinoma. These conditions cause premature death or disability. For these reasons, people who have overweight decide to change their lives, improve health, and increase the possibility of fulfilling themselves in a community. Therefore, this task is not for everyone.

However, everyone knows that weight loss will give you not only a beach-ready body. Weight loss will help improve your health, provide career development and increase your prosperity. In addition, this is only a few reasons for losing weight. Let us see what will bring you DASH diet and weight loss.

1. You will have a beautiful smile and healthy skin. A healthy diet will affect your health and your appearance accordingly. A healthy diet rich in vitamins and minerals will keep your skin smooth and healthy.
2. You will improve the quality of sleep. Excess weight negatively affects the quality of sleep. In the first instance, it is associated with excessive fat in the chest and neck. Excess fat interferes with normal breathing and worsens the heart. You can avoid this situation if you lead an active lifestyle and eat healthy foods.
3. You will improve the quality of vision. Because of excess weight, many people have vision problems. In the first instance, it happens because of increased eye pressure. Therefore, you can improve the quality of vision by reducing weight.
4. You will improve your positions in the ranking of beauty and attractiveness. It is always pleasant to jump from the 70th position of the ranking to the top ten!
5. You will feel more comfortable and confident in a circle of friends, colleagues, and in any other team.
6. You will get physical capabilities (easier to walk, climb stairs, work in the garden to play and run with children).
7. You will get the work of your dreams. It is hard for overweight people to find work. Maybe it is unfair, but it is a fact. Nevertheless, studies confirm that even experience and professionalism are sometimes less important than your weight.

8. You will improve your health and well-being (reduce shortness of breath, reduce high blood pressure, joint pain, spine pain, improve carbohydrate and lipid metabolism).
9. You will be able to buy clothes cheaper! It is no secret that large size clothing is more expensive.
10. Dash diet is a good, easy, safe, and useful approach to losing weight. It is not limited to time. The composition of foods that contain vitamins and trace elements favorably affect the condition of the skin, hair, and nails.

You should agree, for the sake of these pleasant moments should work hard for months or even years! You must try DASH diet. Who knows perhaps and your way of life will radically change to the best for you!

Good luck!

The DASH Dietary Program

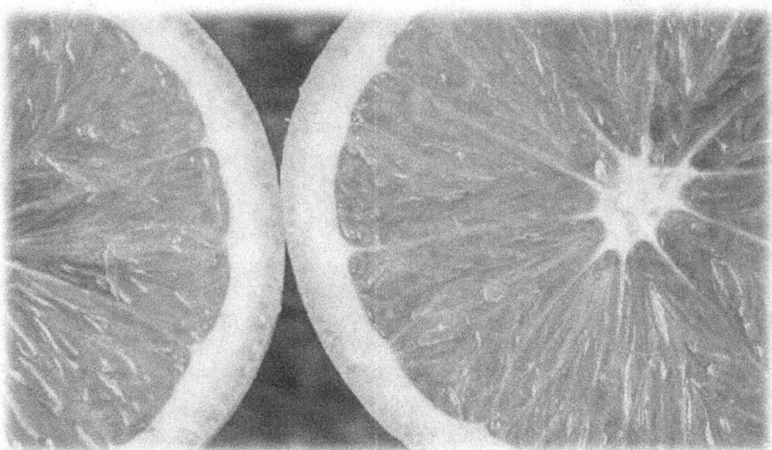

According to the doctors, it is necessary to control not only the use of salt. Many products can differently affect blood pressure and overweight. However, in this case, we are interested in products that will help you normalize blood pressure and replace lose your weight.

A group of American specialists working in the National Institute of Health, as well as in the National Institute of Lung Disease, Heart and Blood, developed and tested a healthy nutrition program designed for people suffering from high blood pressure. The essence of this DASH program may seem very familiar to us. Such a nutrition diet involves the use of foods that do not contain fat, and especially saturated fats.

In addition, the products that are included in the program contain little cholesterol. The diet is focused on eating fresh vegetables, fresh fruits, and healthy dairy products with a reduced percentage of fat. In addition, the program excludes fatty meat, chocolate sweets, and any other sweets. Necessary products are fish, poultry, various nuts and products that are made from whole grains.

Probably, at first glance, it may seem that such a diet is designed for all people with a sick heart because it is very similar to diets that reduce cholesterol. Therefore, you may have a question about the effect on blood pressure indicators, because it is known that both cholesterol and fats cannot influence pressure indices independently.

Indeed, the programs mentioned are very similar, but the DASH program focuses on those foods that have the highest potassium content and magnesium that are rich in calcium. The program is also focused on products with the lowest possible sodium content. These elements can play the most important role in regulating blood pressure indicators. These substances are kind of opponents of sodium, which can weaken its negative aggressive effect on our blood vessels. Actually, therefore, such products need to be consumed quite a lot.

In addition, DASH diet provides your body with potassium, calcium, and magnesium, which acting together have a powerful normalizing effect on blood pressure. Increased consumption of potassium, magnesium, and calcium while limiting the consumption of sodium has a very definite effect on blood pressure. This combination of nutrients acts as a diuretic, which helps the body, eliminate excess salt. In addition, you should avoid fatty, sweet, salty, smoked and canned food. The DASH diet is your conscious choice of vegetarian and natural food. In the first instance, you should determine the number of calories that required for your age and activity level in order to understand how you will spend those calories, and do not forget to limit the intake of salt.

This diet is balanced, which means that the indicators of proteins, fats, and carbohydrates in the diet are close to the value of the norm. This is especially important for people suffering from hypertension people. Dash offers a varied and tasty menu, which can be modified at will! Most importantly, follow the general rules of daily portions. With time, if you want, you can go to vegetarian food. The diet is designed so that in any case will be effective.

The Dash diet also provides some strict prohibitions, which, however, do not differ from the prohibitions of most diet programs: no fast food, confectionery products and sweets, roast, smoked and salty foods.

Let us look at the key principles of the diet:
- the calorie content of a daily diet should be in the range of 2000-2500 kcal;
- obligatory it is necessary to reduce the daily norm of salt to 2/3 of a teaspoon for healthy people and up to 1/3 of a teaspoon for hypertensive people;
- the main products are meat, fish, vegetables, fruits, and cereals;
- be sure to regularly add to the daily menu whole wheat bread, dairy products with a low-fat content, and dishes containing legumes;
- adipose is limited in favor of vegetable oil;
- it is necessary to give up the use of alcohol and tobacco;
- exclude from the diet of sweets, smoked products, pickles, fatty foods, canned fish, and meat;
- you should increase the intake of products containing potassium, calcium, in magnesium.

The use of Dash diet for weight loss is confirmed both by scientists and by the opinions of the people who chose it. A special effect of weight loss is achieved by combining diet with aerobic exercise. Medical studies of the Dash diet confirm a weight loss of 8-9 kilograms over a four-month period. Without physical activity, weight loss was less. This means that in addition to Dash diet experts recommend an active lifestyle.

Balanced DASH healthy diet can get rid of many diseases or prevent them. You will be able to stabilize your weight effortlessly and restore physical and mental energy. As a result, you will receive good health, which promotes excellent health, beautiful appearance and achieve their goals in life. I think you also should try this popular worldwide nutrition system.

The healthy DASH diet is one of the best diet treatment, which applies to patients with high blood pressure or overweight problems. In addition to regulating the pressure, the DASH diet solves several important problems, namely, the healthy diet reduces enhanced the concentration of cholesterol, prevent some types of cancer, heart disease and stroke, renal gravel, and reduces the risk of developing diabetes. The DASH diet significantly reduces overweight, improves health and quality of life of people. The healthy diet is admitted as one of the best nutrition approaches to the prevention and treatment of diabetes and one of the most effective in diseases of the heart.

Take care and be healthy!

Why the DASH Diet Truly Works for Weight Loss and Blood Pressure

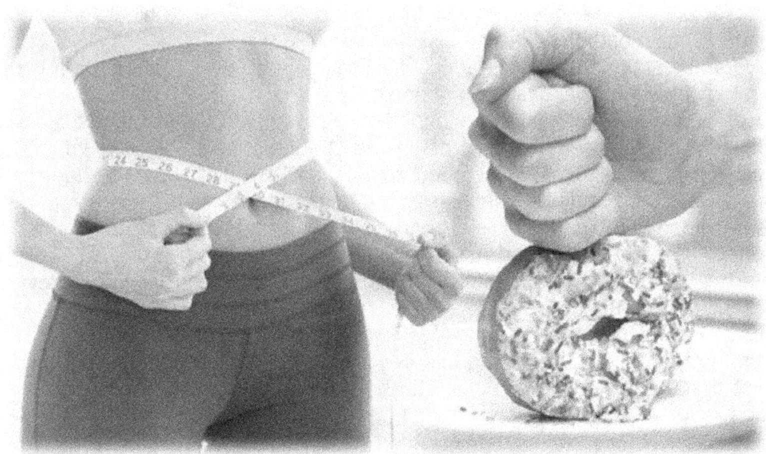

The idea of the DASH diet originated in the United States 20 years ago. Specialists and cardiologists concerned about the growing number of people suffering from high blood pressure. They decided to create a special diet to treat hypertension without pills. The result of five years of work of scientists was a new concept the DASH diet (Dietary Approaches to Stop Hypertension). As it turned out also new diet helps to lose overweight! Moreover, we all know that high blood pressure and overweight are interrelated. People, who followed the DASH diet, were able to maintain the blood pressure parameters and their weight! Thus, a therapeutic diet was in the center of attention of thousands of ordinary people who would like to improve your health and lose weight comfortably and without harm to health.

The healthy DASH diet is a food based on vegetables, fruits, foods rich in potassium and magnesium. Vegetable fiber, vitamins, and minerals have a good effect on the functioning of the cardiovascular system of a human. This is why you should definitely include in the diet such products like sour-milk products, rice, nuts, currants, whole grains, and fresh herbs.

The dietary nutrition of a person with hypertension and the desire to lose weight is based on regularity and split meals. If you have hypertension disease, you need to eat at least 5 times a day, and at the same time, you should observe regular intervals between meals. The last meal should be finished 2 hours before bedtime. It is better to schedule and eat according to your schedule. It is important not only to reduce the size of the portion but also to rationally distribute the consumption of daily calories.

Weight loss is not an easy task. However, any person can lose it if desired. Understanding the changes that occur in your body during this period will undoubtedly help to achieve the best results. Following a healthy diet, you can lose up to 10 kg of excess weight per month. The effectiveness of a diet designed specifically for the prevention of hypertension is able to reduce blood pressure significantly and weight due to the following processes:

1. Reducing the amount of salt in the diet stimulates the removal of excess fluid from the body, reducing blood pressure on the walls of the vessels;
2. The lack of fatty foods reduces the level of cholesterol and improves the blood composition and significantly reduces the weight of a person;

3. The lack of strong tea, coffee, alcohol reduce the burden on the cardiovascular system of a person;
4. At first, you can lose a lot of weight, and then the process starts to slow down. The reason lies in the fact that in the first place the body loses water, and then lose fat.
5. Potassium and magnesium strengthen blood vessels, dilute blood, and reduce the risk of spasm of the vessels.
6. Systematic sports exercises effectively reduce your weight and have a good effect on the cardiovascular system of a person.

Developed by the National Institute for the U.S. nutrition plan can lead to a lowering of blood pressure after 2 weeks from the beginning of adherence to the DASH diet. Based on the results of clinical trials, researchers found that the DASH diet system besides controlling blood pressure could bring other benefits to the health of the patient, namely, to prevent or slow the development of osteoporosis, heart disease, diabetes of the 2nd type and cancer. In this regard, the American Heart Association recommends the use of DASH diet not only for primary and secondary prevention of arterial hypertension and for prevention of cardiovascular diseases.

Especially effective adherence to DASH diet for lowering blood pressure in the elderly age group, however, if you become a follower of the DASH diet-eating plan at a young age this means that the development of hypertension can be avoided altogether.

Good luck!

The Importance of Exercises

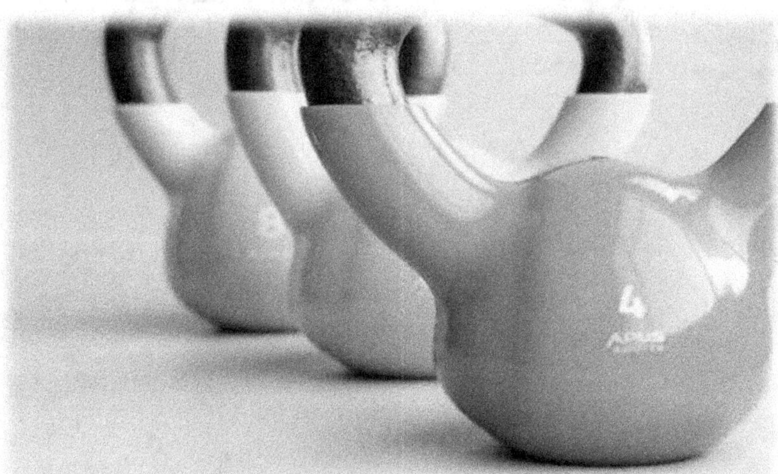

Exercises and active lifestyle speed up metabolic process, oxygenate the cells, accelerate the lymph flow and circulation, improve digestion and help to eliminate toxins from the body through sweat. This is the ideal set of factors needed to reduce weight. In addition, exercises will help you lose weight, strengthen your muscles, increases immunity, improve the cardiovascular system, stimulate the production of a hormone of joy, and increase the level of endurance and strength of your body. There are the most effective sports that will help you quickly achieve the desired result. Let us discuss each of them.

Swimming. One of the most effective sports that helps to correct your figure. 1 hour of swimming will allow you to burn off up to 600 calories if you follow all the rules. You can swim with a trainer who will monitor the quality of the exercises and the process of weight reduction. Before the swim, you need to do a warm-up because it will help to avoid spasms and injuries.

Dancing. Perhaps, this is one of the most interesting sports with its bright varieties. One hour of training can burn off up to 500 calories and get many positive impressions. For girls, such weight loss will be especially pleasant, because they not only correct their figure but also realize their creativity.

Bicycle riding. This is the most effective method for those who want to correct the shape of the thighs and buttocks. You should ride a bicycle for only 30 minutes 3 times a week. In a month, you will notice how the excess weight disappears, and the muscles become elastic and elastic.

Run. There are different running techniques that help to lose weight. During running, you can burn off up to 750 calories in just 30 minutes. However, to achieve such results, you should do this kind of sport under the supervision of an instructor. Otherwise, you can get problems with muscles and joints.

Fitness. Rhythmic exercises are designed specifically to make your body ideal. Exercises suggest cardiac and anaerobic exercises, which combine to affect fat burning and the formation of strong muscles. As a rule, classes last for 1 hour, and you need to visit them 3 times a week.

Aerobics. This sport is designed specifically for weight loss. It combines complex exercises and dance elements, which makes training more diverse and interesting. In one lesson, you can lose up to 400 calories, which is an excellent indicator.

Even the most active workouts will not give the desired results if you do not comply with some rules of losing weight. Any sport should be combined with a balanced DASH diet. You should follow all the recommendations of coaches or instructors. In addition, you should remember that training should be regular because it is the only way to lose weight consistently.

Good luck!

HEALTHY BREAKFAST

Omelet with chicken breast

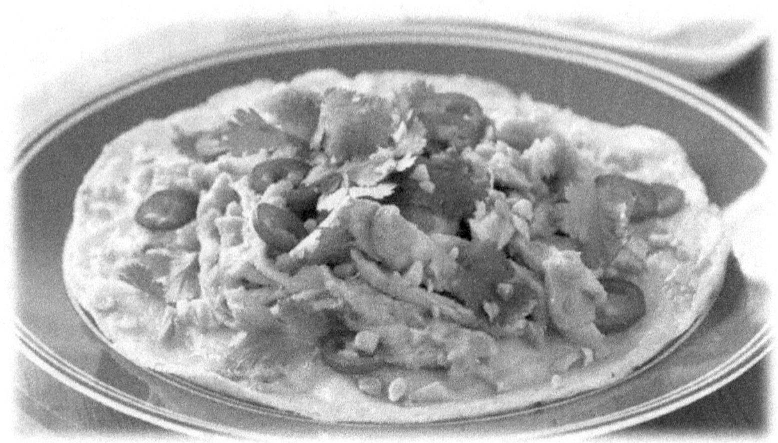

Ingredients (7 servings):

- 2 eggs
- 100 g of boiled chicken fillet
- 1 tomato
- 1 carrot
- 1 onion
- 2 teaspoons of olive oil
- spices to taste

Cooking instruction:

In the first instance, you should heat the olive oil in a pan and lightly fry the chopped onions, tomatoes and carrots. You should be divided the meat into pieces. Then you should randomly lay the sliced meat and add spices to taste. In addition, beat up the eggs and add a little salt. Stir well and pour into the frying pan. You should reduce the heat to a minimum, and cover the frying pan with a lid. The omelet should be cooked no more than 6-8 minutes. Well done!

Bon Appetite!

Scrambled eggs with vegetables

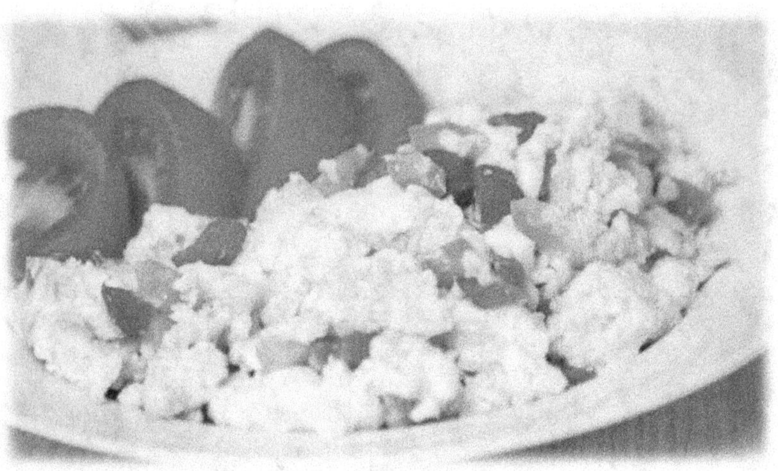

Ingredients (5 servings):

- 4 eggs
- 2 fresh sweet pepper
- 1 onion
- 2 medium-sized tomatoes
- fresh herbs to taste

Cooking instruction:

In the first instance, you should oil and preheat a frying pan. After that, whisk the eggs in a deep bowl. Then chop one fresh sweet pepper, onion and tomatoes. Next, you should add the chopped vegetables to the whisked eggs. Now mix the mass thoroughly. When the frying pan is heated, you should pour the egg mass into the frying pan. Cook for 15 minutes. Do not forget to decorate the scrambled eggs with fresh herbs to your taste. Well done! Serve immediately!

Bon Appetite!

Italian frittata with vegetables

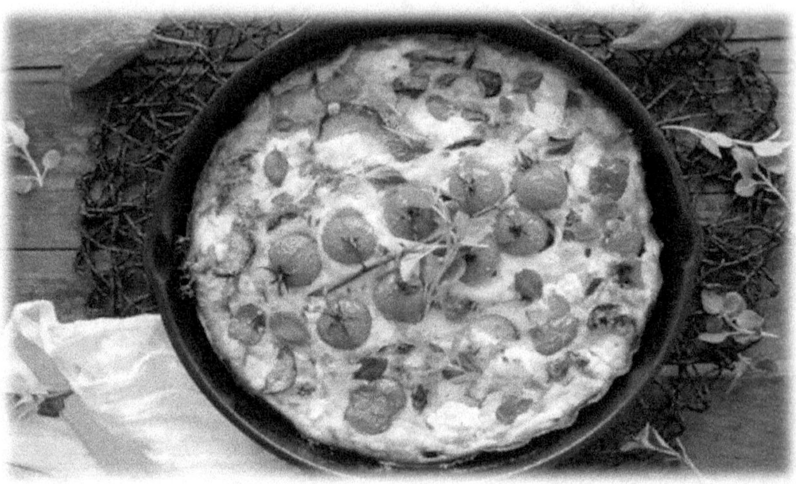

Ingredients (9 servings):

- 4 eggs
- 1 tomato
- 1 sweet pepper
- 1 onion
- 1 clove of garlic
- 1 bunch of parsley
- olive oil
- basil dried
- black pepper to taste

Cooking instruction:

In the first instance, you should chop the fresh parsley. Then beat the eggs. Stir eggs with chopped parsley. Leave the egg mixture for 5 minutes. At this time, you should fry the garlic in olive oil. Then add chopped onion, garlic, tomato and cook for another five minutes. Add the egg mixture and fry until the eggs are ready. After that, place the dish in the oven and bake until cooked at a temperature of 180 C. This will take about 15 minutes. Then add pepper to taste. Do not forget to decorate the frittata with a dry basil. Well done!

Bon Appetite!

Pie with carrots and cheese

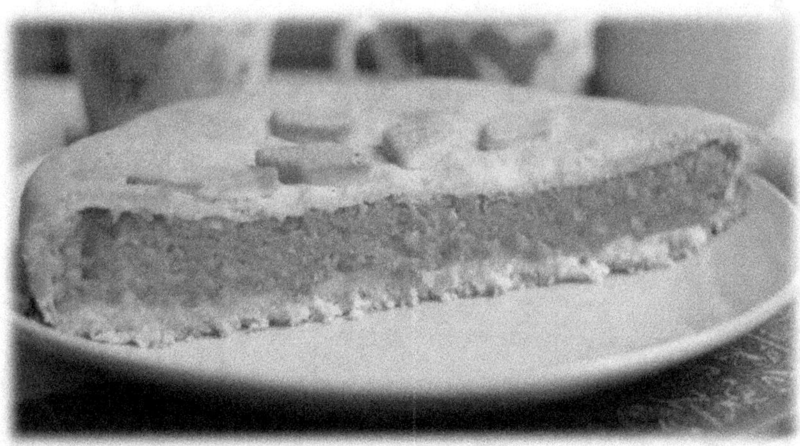

Ingredients (5 servings):

- 1½ cups of grated carrots
- ½ cup of yellow bell pepper
- 8 large eggs
- pepper to taste
- 12 teaspoons of grated cheese

Cooking instruction

In the first instance, you should preheat the oven to 190 °C. After that, oil the silicone mold for baking pie. Then put the grated carrots and pepper in a large bowl. You should stir it well. Pour about 3 tablespoons of the vegetable mixture into the baking mold. Then you should fill the mold in 2/3. After that, it is necessary to whisk two eggs in a separate bowl. Add pepper to taste. Next, you should pour 2-3 tablespoons of the egg mixture into the mold. After that, you should fill the mold in ¾. Then put grated cheese on top of the mold and bake for 18-20 minutes until a golden crust appears. Well done!

Bon Appetite!

Egg rolls with vegetables

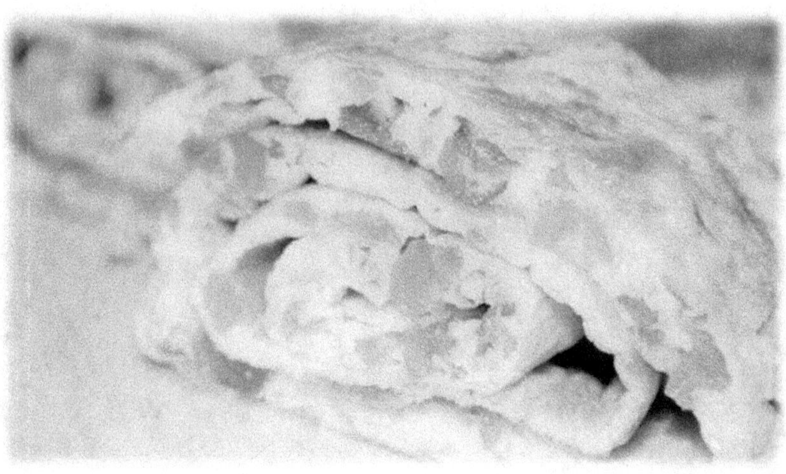

Ingredients (5 servings):

- 4 eggs
- black pepper to taste
- 100 g of any herbs
- 1 carrot
- vegetable oil
- 1 red pepper
- 100 g of boiled mushrooms

Cooking instruction:

In the first instance, you should beat the eggshell and pour the contents into a deep bowl. Then you should finely chop the fresh herbs, red pepper, boiled mushrooms, and carrots. Stir the egg mixture thoroughly with chopped vegetables. After that, you should add pepper to taste. Stir the egg mixture thoroughly again. Pour a quarter of the egg mixture into a heated and oiled frying pan. If you see that the egg pancake is cooked, then you should roll it. Repeat the same steps with the whole egg mixture. The cooked rolls cut into small pieces. Well done!

Bon Appetite!

Cauliflower with cream cheese and chicken

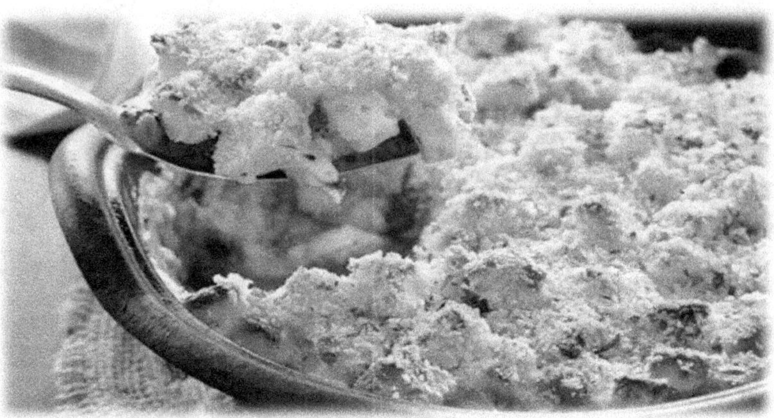

Ingredients (7 servings):

- 900 g of cauliflower
- 1 white onion
- 1 tablespoon of butter
- 120 g of cream cheese
- 120 ml of fatty cream
- 60 ml of chicken broth
- 1 tablespoon of grated cheese

Cooking instruction

In the first instance, you should cut cauliflower into small pieces. Then put them in a saucepan with lightly salted water and cook on a medium heat for 20-30 minutes until they become soft and tender. Throw the vegetable in a colander and set it aside. Take a deep frying pan and melt butter on it. You should fry sliced white onions in the melted butter. Cook on a medium heat until the onion becomes soft. Then put cooked cauliflower on the bottom of the frying pan. After that, mix it with the onion. Next, chop the parts of cauliflower into smaller pieces. Reduce the heat and pour chicken broth and cream into the frying pan. Mix thoroughly. Then, add the cream cheese to the mixture. Stir the ingredients until the cheese has melted. If the contents of the frying pan are too thick, you can pour broth. Finally, sprinkle the contents of grated cheese and mix. After that, remove the frying pan from the heat. Now you should preheat the oven to about 160°C. Place the cauliflower along with the cream sauce into the baking dish, and sprinkle with grated cheese on top. You should bake for 15-20 minutes. Well done!

Bon Appetite!

Oatmeal with berries and muesli

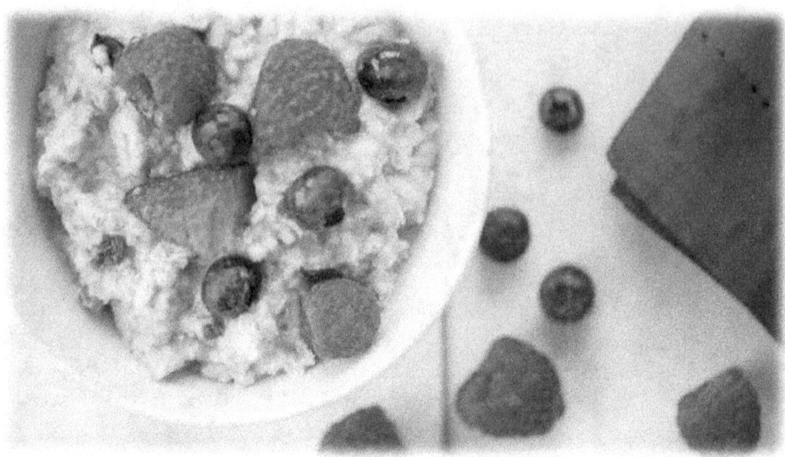

Ingredients (6 servings):

- 2 cups of oatmeal
- 3 cups of low-fat milk or water
- 20 g of butter
- fresh berries to taste
- muesli to taste
- dried fruits to taste

Cooking instruction:

In the first instance, you should bring the low-fat milk or water to a boil. After that, add the oatmeal and mix the mass thoroughly. You should cook the oatmeal, not more than for 5-7 minutes on a low heat. The oatmeal should become thick and homogeneous. Do not forget to stir the mass constantly. Then remove oatmeal from the heat, and add 20 g of butter. Stir well. Add berries, muesli and dried fruits to taste. In addition, you can add some fresh fruits. For example, apples, pear, kiwi etc. Well done!
Bon Appetite!

Granola bar with cocoa and coconut

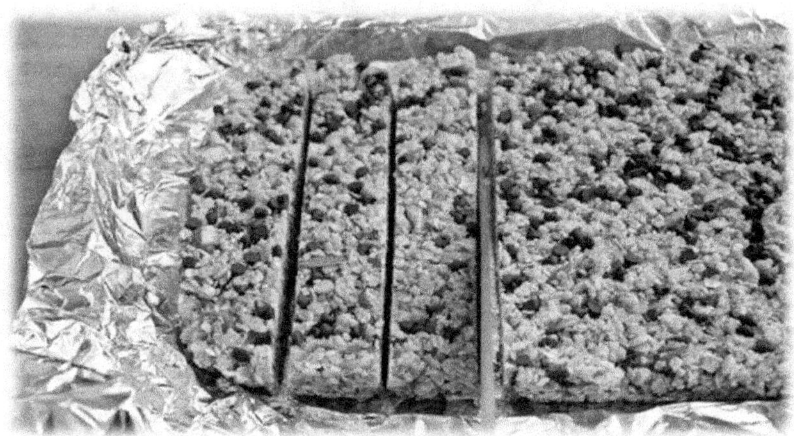

Ingredients (9 servings):

- 1 ½ cup of almonds
- 1 ½ cups of different nuts and grains
- 1 glass of flax seeds
- 1 cup of coconut flakes
- ¼ cup of sugar substitute
- ½ teaspoon of salt
- ¼ cup of coconut oil
- 1 egg
- ½ cup of cocoa beans

Cooking instruction

In the first instance, you should preheat the oven to 150°C and cover a large dripping pan with a parchment. Then mix almonds, remaining nuts, and grains in a blender. Stir until the mixture looks like crumbs. Now you can place the mixture into a large bowl. After that, you should add flax seeds, coconut flakes, sugar substitute, and salt. Then sprinkle with coconut oil and mix. After that, you should add eggs and stir well. The mixture should be homogeneous. Next, you should add the cocoa beans and then place the mixture in the dripping pan and bake it for 20 minutes. Do not forget stirring constantly. Well done!

Bon Appetite!

Cheesecake with lemon and cream cheese

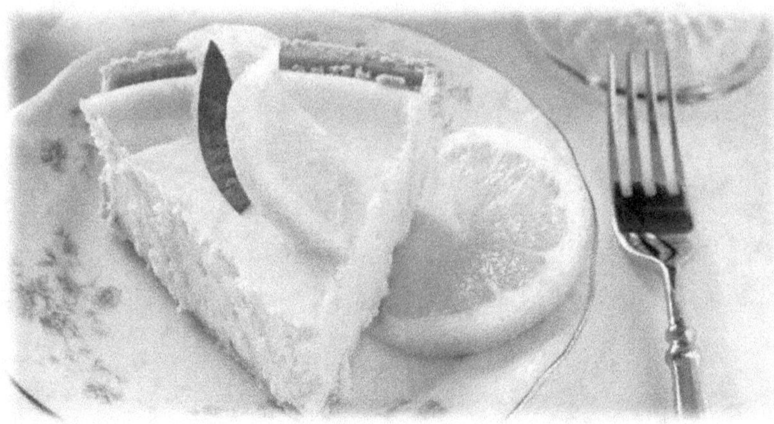

Ingredients (6 servings):

- 200 g of soft cream cheese
- 50 ml of fatty cream
- 1 teaspoon of stevia (liquid)
- 1 soup spoon of lemon juice
- vanillin to taste
- ¼ teaspoon of lemon peel

Cooking instruction

This is a dessert of cold cooking. Therefore, the process of cooking of this dessert will take only five minutes. In the first instance, you should put the cheese and cream in a deep bowl. Mix the ingredients with each other by a mixer until the consistency becomes like a pudding. Then you should add stevia, lemon juice, vanillin, and zest. Thoroughly mix the mass. Spread mass on the dessert bowls. After that, put the dessert in the fridge for 1 to 2 hours. Well done! Serve immediately!

Bon Appetite!

Smoothies with chokeberry, apple, and banana

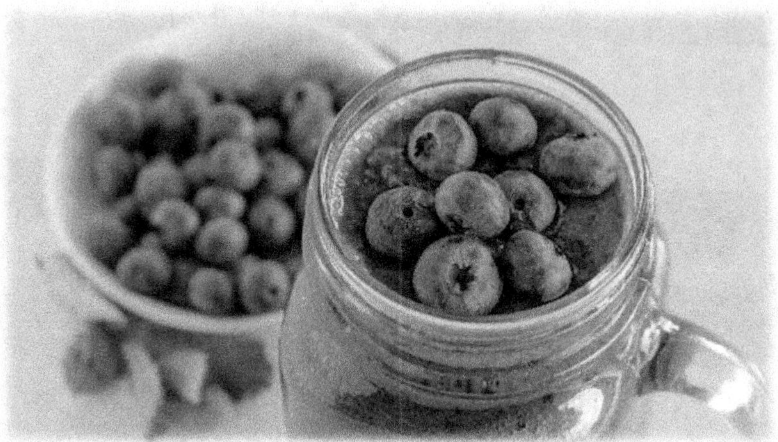

Ingredients (6 servings):

- 100 g of chokeberry
- 2 apples
- 1 large banana
- 100 ml of water
- 1 tablespoons honey
- pinch of ground cinnamon

Cooking instruction:

In the first instance, you should cut the apples in half, and then carefully remove the seeds. Then cut the halves of the fruit into several pieces so that they quickly and finely grind. Next, you should peel a banana and cut it into rings. After, mix the cut fruits in a blender. After that, you can add the black chokeberry. Then add a little cold filtered water to make the smoothies more fluid. For flavor, you should add a pinch of ground cinnamon to the ingredients. Then mix all the ingredients in the blender. Now you can pour the fresh smoothies into glasses and decorate with chokeberry and a stick of cinnamon.

Bon Appetite!

Smoothies with pumpkin, apple, and banana

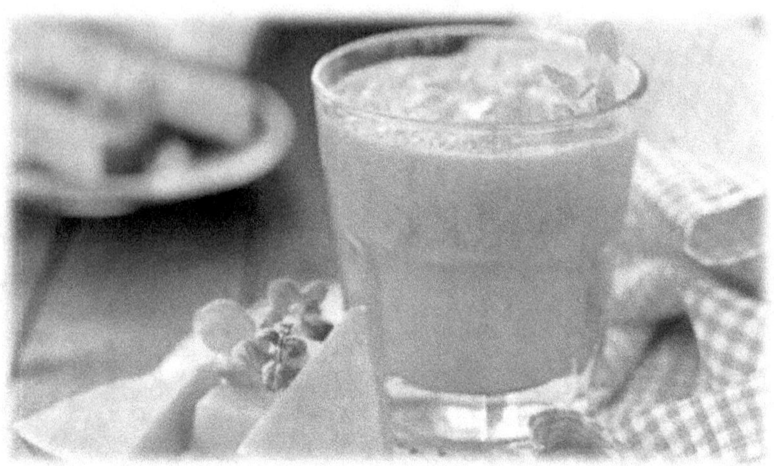

Ingredients (5 servings):

- 300 g of pumpkin
- 1 large sweet apple
- 1 large banana
- 300 ml of yogurt
- 1 tablespoon sesame seeds

Cooking instruction:

In the first instance, you should cut the pumpkin into small cubes. Move them to the bowl of the blender for grinding. Banana clean and, as usual, cut into pieces. Add the banana pieces to the pumpkin. Cut the apple in half, and cut out the core. Cut the halves of the apple into pieces of medium size and add to the components. Mix everything in a blender. Fruit with pumpkin should become a homogeneous and thick mass. Add the yogurt. Mix the mixture again with a blender so that the cocktail becomes liquid. Seeds of sesame fry in a pan, stirring constantly for 30 seconds. Then pour the seeds into a dry plate so that the seeds cool down a little. Pour the ready smoothies into tall glasses and decorate with sesame seeds.

Bon Appetite!

HEALTHY LUNCHES

Pancakes with spinach and cottage cheese

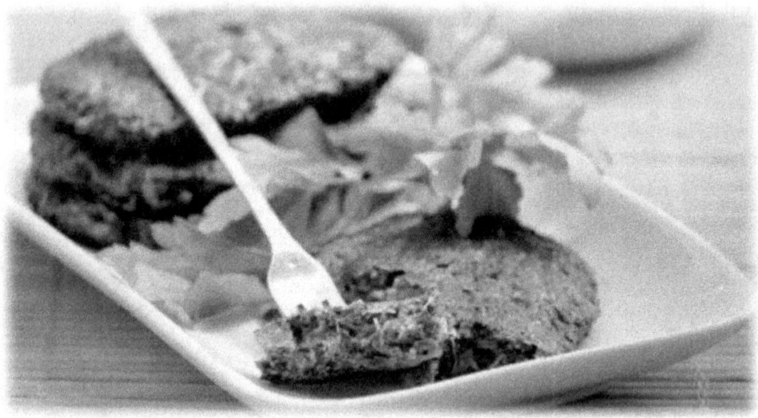

Ingredients (6 servings):

- 200 g of spinach
- 50 g of oatmeal
- 2 g of cheese
- 100 g of cheese
- 2 eggs
- black pepper to taste

Cooking instruction:

In the first instance, you should finely chop the fresh spinach and cook in boiling water 5 minutes. Then drain the boiling water and leave the spinach to cool. After that, you should chop the spinach, oatmeal, grated cheese, eggs and cottage cheese in a blender. Now, heat 1 tablespoon of olive oil in a frying pan and bake pancakes until ready. Well done! Serve pancakes hot with fresh lettuce and vegetables.

Bon Appetite!

Zucchini Lasagna with mixed cheeses

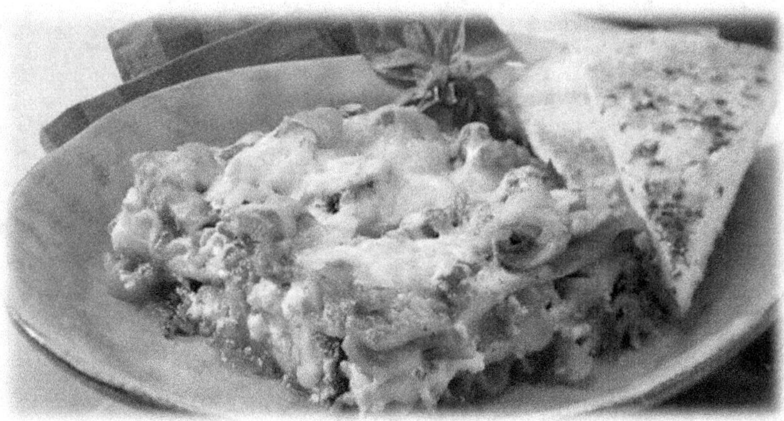

Ingredients (10 servings):

- 500 g of beef
- 1 ½ teaspoons black pepper
- 1 tablespoon of olive oil
- a large egg
- 1 chopped onion
- 4 cloves of garlic
- 3 crushed tomatoes
- chopped basil
- 3 zucchinis
- 1 ½ cups of ricotta,
- 4 cups of grated Mozzarella cheese
- ¼ cup of Parmigiano Reggiano

Cooking instruction

In the first instance, you should cook the beef in a pan. After cooking the beef, use a colander to drain the water. Next, add olive oil to the pan. Place there the chopped garlic and onion. Cook vegetables with the beef for 1.5 minutes. Keep in mind that you should place the tomatoes, basil, and black pepper to the beef and cook all the ingredients for 35 minutes. In addition, you should fry both sides of sliced zucchini for 3 minutes in the pan. Then preheat the oven to approximately 180°C. After that, mix Ricotta, egg, and Parmesan in the same dish thoroughly. Pour ½ cup of sauce on the bottom of the pan. Next, cover the sauce layer with a layer of fried zucchini and add ½ cup of ricotta cheese mixture. The next layer is mozzarella cheese. The last layer you should cover with foil. You should bake all layers for 30 minutes. After opening the foil and bake for 25 minutes. Then place add mozzarella and bake for 10 minutes. Well done! Serve immediately!

Bon Appetite!

Broccoli cream soup

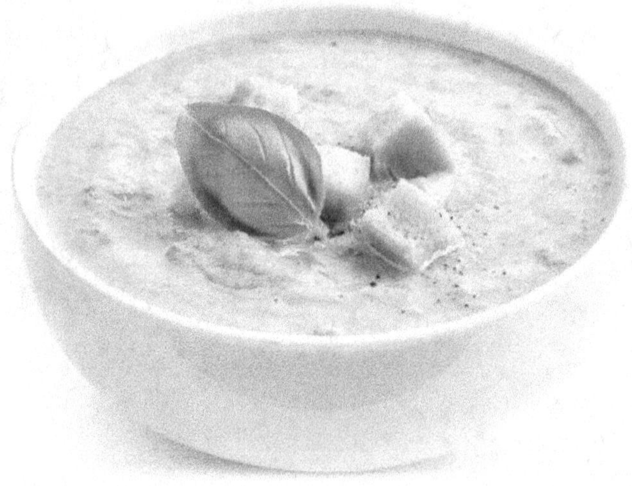

Ingredients (6 servings):

- 400 g of broccoli
- 1 tablespoon of grated cheese
- 200 ml of low-fat cream
- 1 teaspoon of butter
- 1 white onions
- 1l of chicken broth

Cooking instruction:

In the first instance, you should melt the butter in the frying pan. Then slice the onion and fry it. Slices of onion should become golden and soft. After that, add the chicken broth to the frying pan. You should cook on a medium heat until the broth boils. Now, you can add chopped broccoli. Then the content should boil again. After that, reduce the heat. Cook the soup until the broccoli becomes soft. After that, you can remove the frying pan from the heat. All the ingredients should be placed in the blender for grinding. Well done! Next, you should add to the ground ingredients low-fat cream and grated cheese. Mix the mass with help of blender again. The soup should be served immediately.

Bon Appetite!

Cream soup with chickpeas and pumpkin

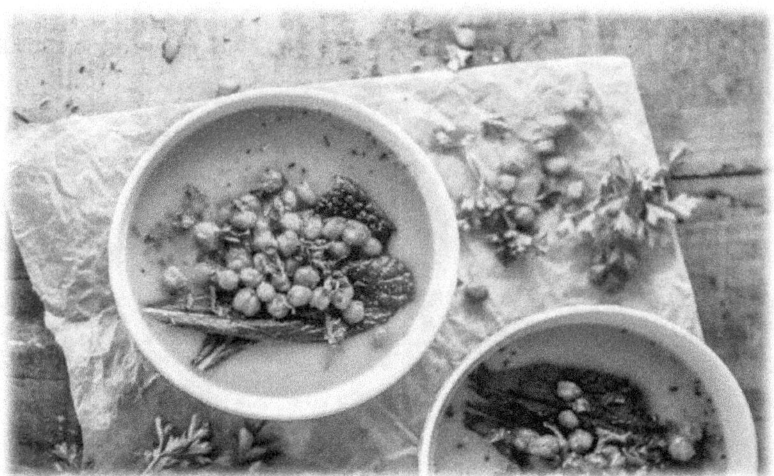

Ingredients (8 servings):

- 100 g of chickpeas
- 4 potatoes
- 3 carrots
- 1 onion
- 50 g of pumpkin
- fresh herbs
- pepper to taste
- olive oil

Cooking instruction:

The cup of chickpeas must be placed in a glass of water for the night. For one cup of chickpeas, you should use four cups of water. After that, you should cook the chickpeas about half an hour. Cut the pumpkin into cubes and add to the chickpeas. Then add the chopped potatoes, onions and carrots. You should boil the vegetables until they become soft. After that, you should put the contents of the pan into a blender and grind well all the ingredients. Now, you can add the olive oil and pepper to taste. Next, you should cook the soup for another 10 minutes. Well done!

Bon Appetite!

Cream- soup with vegetables

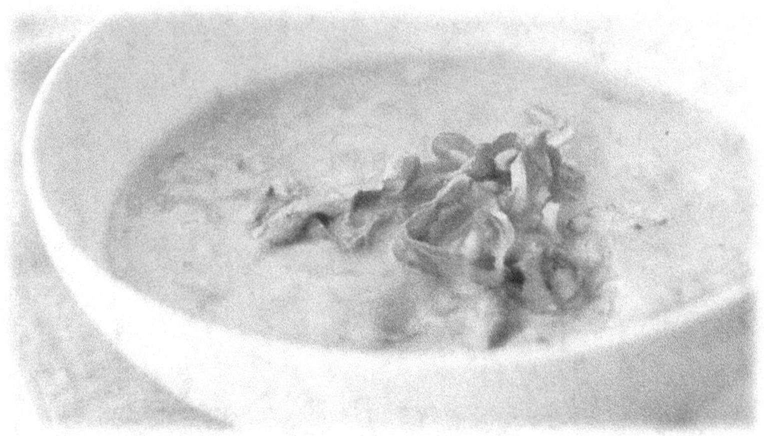

Ingredients (13 servings):

- 2 tablespoons of butter
- 2 cloves of garlic
- 1 onion
- 2 carrots
- 1 celery
- ¼ cup of flour
- 4 cups of chicken broth

- 1 cup of milk
- grated low-fat cheese
- cauliflower
- a bay leaf
- black pepper to taste
- fresh herbs to taste

Cooking instruction:

In the first instance, you should chop all vegetables. Add the chopped onion, carrots, celery and garlic to the melted butter in the frying pan. Mix the vegetables thoroughly. Then add cauliflower and a bay leaf. Now, you can add the flour to the vegetables. In one minute, a brown color should appear. In addition, you should add the chicken broth and milk. Mix the mass intensively. The broth should be thick. You should cook on a medium heat for 15 minutes until the cauliflower becomes soft. Then pepper to taste. If the broth is too thick, you can add milk. Well done! Do not forget to decorate your cream-soup with fresh herbs and grated cheese.

Bon Appetite!

Chicken baked with spinach

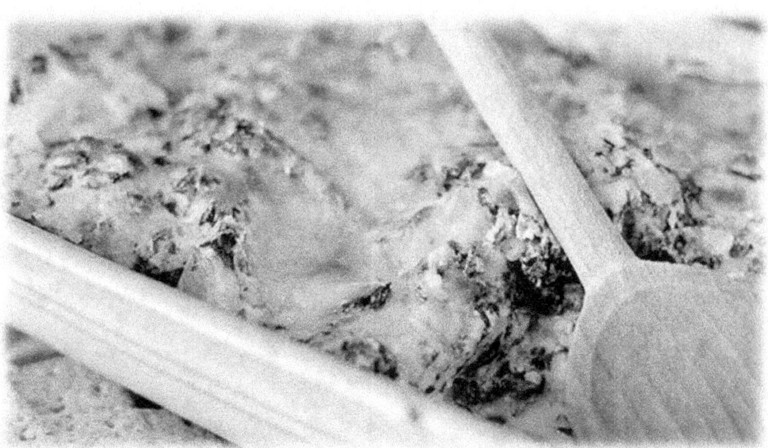

Ingredients (8 servings):

- 500 g of chicken fillet
- 250 g of spinach
- 1 onion
- 200 ml of low-fat sour cream
- 100 g of grated cheese
- 3 tablespoons of vegetable oil
- pepper to taste
- spices to taste

Cooking instruction:

In the first instance, you should cut the chicken fillet into pieces. Then add pepper and spices, such as sweet paprika, ginger, etc. Then fry chopped onion. After that add the spinach, sour cream, and pepper to taste. Stir well. You should cook on medium heat until the cream thickens. You can also add chopped garlic and a pinch of hot pepper. Now, place the chicken in a heat-resistant form, and add the spinach and grated cheese. You should roast the meat for 15 minutes at a temperature of 190 °C. Well done!

Bon Appetite!

Vegetables baked in foil

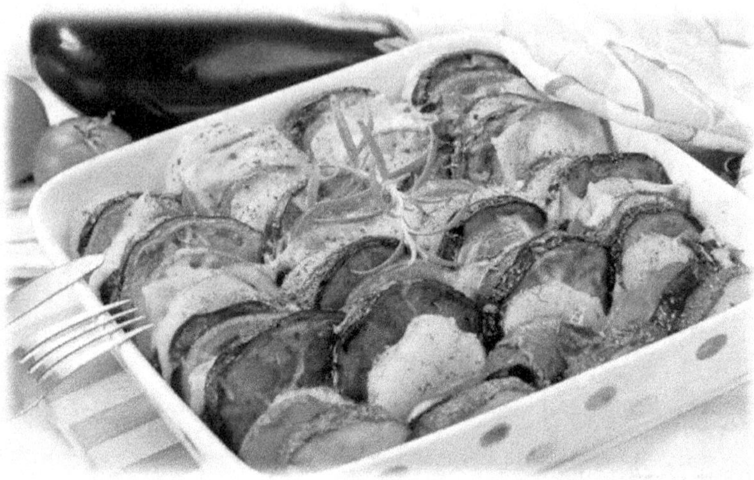

Ingredients (11 servings):

- 1 eggplant
- 1 vegetable marrow
- 400 g of sweet pepper
- 250 g of tomatoes
- 1 carrot
- 100 g of champignons

- 1 onion
- 1 clove of garlic
- 1 chili pepper
- parsley to taste
- 6 tablespoons of vegetable oil

Cooking instruction:

In the first instance, you should cut the eggplant in circles no more than one cm thick. Then you should cut the vegetable marrow into pieces no longer than four cm. Also, cut the carrots into pieces of the same size as vegetable marrow. After that, you should remove the seeds of sweet pepper and cut it into large pieces. Now you can cut the champignons into halves. The onion should be cut into thick rings. Then chop garlic and parsley. Mix all the ingredients, except tomatoes, with a lot of vegetable oil and a tablespoon of salt. Add the chili pepper. You should pickle vegetables in oil with salt and spices for at least an hour, and preferably one and a half to two hours. Do not forget to mix vegetables thoroughly every half an hour. Then drain excess liquid. Then you should heat the oven to 300°C. Marinated vegetables put on a baking sheet over the foil layer. Add the tomatoes. If the tomatoes are large, they can be cut into halves or quarters. Cover the vegetables with foil and bake for 15 minutes. Then open the foil and bake the vegetables for a few more minutes. Well done!
Bon Appetite!

Soup with spinach and salmon

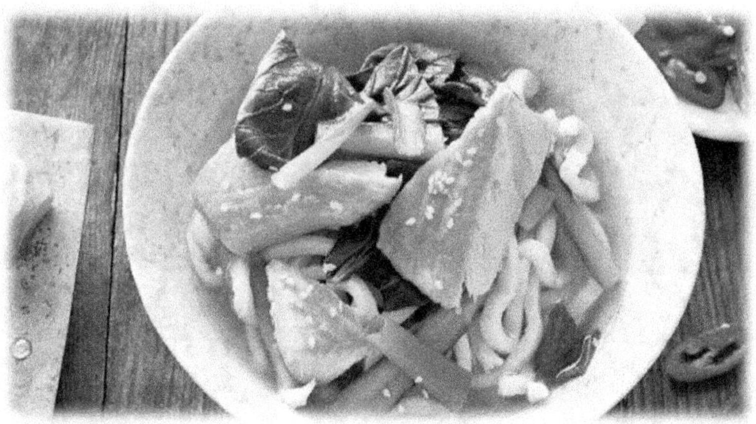

Ingredients (9 servings):

- 400 g of salmon (you can also add squids to your taste)
- 100 g spinach
- 1 red pepper
- 1 carrot
- 1 onion
- 1 teaspoon paprika
- black pepper to taste
- vegetable oil

Cooking instruction:

In the first instance, you should put the fish in the casserole. Add cold water, and then put the casserole on the fire. After boiling water, you should clear the broth from the foam. After this, it is necessary to cook the broth on low heat for 20-25 minutes. Remove the bones from the boiled fish, and then divide the meat into medium-sized pieces. After chop the onion, red pepper and carrots into small cubes. Sliced vegetables fry in vegetable oil. Then place the vegetables in the broth and bring the soup to a boil. Boil all the ingredients for 10 to 12 minutes. Then add the chopped spinach to the pan with the fish pieces. Add pepper to taste. Stir the broth thoroughly and add the paprika. Bring the broth to a boil. In addition, in two minutes after boiling, you should remove the casserole from the heat. Well done!
Bon Appetite!

Fish broth with spices

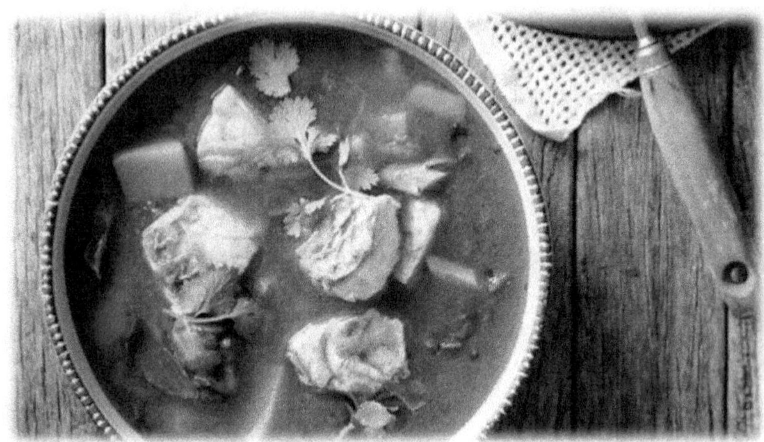

Ingredients (10 servings):

- 400 g of any fish
- 1 onion
- 1 lemon
- 4 tablespoons of olive oil
- 10 g of bay leaves
- 1 hot pepper
- 1 clove of garlic
- herbs, such as thyme, dill, or coriander
- ginger ground to taste

Cooking instruction:

In the first instance, you should cut the fish into large pieces. Then you should clean the onion. Place the onions in a saucepan with boiling water, and add spices, chopped herbs, and hot pepper. Stir the broth thoroughly. Then add olive oil to taste. You should cook the broth for 10 minutes. Add the fish and cook for another 10 minutes. Remove the boiled fish and herbs from the saucepan. The fish should cool down, and then remove the bones from the meat. Then place the meat of fish and garlic in the broth. Now you should add lemon juice. Well done!

Bon Appetite!

Baked seafood with vegetables and lemon

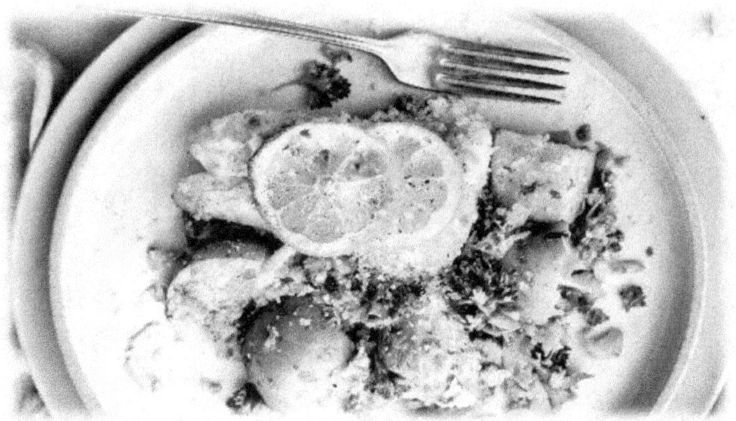

Ingredients (12 servings):

- 50 g of butter
- 2 carrots
- 1/2 of lemon (peel and juice)
- 3-4 sprigs of chopped dill
- black pepper to taste
- 30 g of soy sauce
- laurel leaf to taste
- 2 tomatoes
- 2 onions
- 30 g of lemon juice
- 500 g of seafood
- 5 tablespoons of vegetable oil

Cooking instruction

In the first instance, you should defrost the seafood by placing them on the top shelf of the refrigerator. Grate the carrot and cut the onion into cubes. Then a little salt and fry in vegetable oil for 10-12 minutes until the appearance of golden color. After that, you should cut the tomatoes and lemon into circles. Put tomatoes on the foil, then carrots and onions. On top of the layer of vegetables, put seafood, sprigs of dill and 2-3 circles of lemon. Add the bay leaves and black pepper to taste. Do not forget to melt the butter and mix it with lemon juice and soy sauce. Add the mixture to vegetables and seafood. Tightly wrap the envelope from the foil and place it in the oven. Bake in the oven for 10-12 minutes. Well done!

Bon Appetite!

Baked salmon with herbs

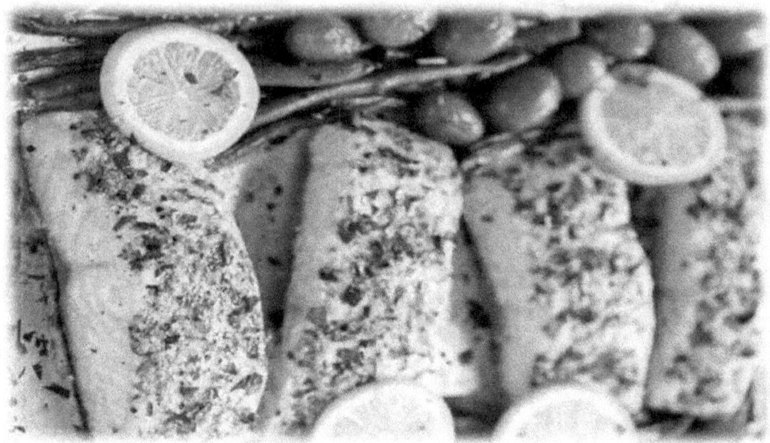

Ingredients (4 servings):

- fresh frames of salmon
- 4 cloves of garlic
- black pepper to taste
- any herbs you want
- any spices for fish
- grated cheese

Cooking instruction

In the first instance, you should preheat the oven to approximately 200°C. Add pepper to the frames of salmon. After that put fresh garlic on a sheet of foil. Do not oil the foil with sunflower oil! The fish should be baked in its own juice and herbs. The peppered frames of salmon you should put on the layer of garlic. In addition, you can use any herbs, for example, dill, parsley, green onions, basil, coriander. Now the salmon is ready for baking. Sprinkle with previously grated cheese the frames of salmon. Tightly wrap the fish in the foil and place it in the oven. Reduce the heat to 150 ° C. Bake for 20 minutes. Well done!

Bon Appetite!

Trout baked with tomatoes

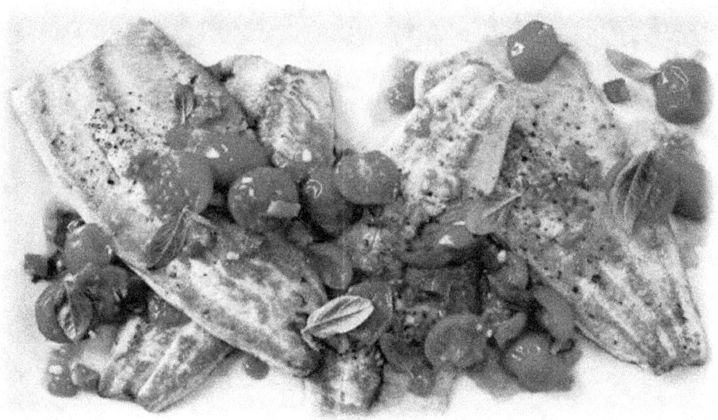

Ingredients (9 servings):

- 1 kg of trout
- 100 g onion green
- 500 g cherry tomatoes
- 1 lemon
- 4 sprigs of thyme
- a couple of sprigs of parsley
- 2 tablespoons olive oil
- black pepper to taste
- spices for fish to taste

Cooking instruction

In the first instance, you should remove the scales, the umbles, and gills. After that, you should wash the fish under running water, and dry with a paper towel. Place a piece of foil on the counter. Then oil the foil with olive oil. If you are afraid that the fish will still attach to the foil during baking, cut the onions with rings and place it on the foil, and then lay the fish on the onion layer. Sprinkle the fish with olive oil. Add pepper, and spices to the fish outside and inside the trout. Leave the fish for a few minutes to marinate. Stuff the fish with a sprig of parsley, a couple of twigs of thyme, green onions, cherry tomatoes and lemon. Bake in preheated oven to 180 degrees for 20 minutes. Well done! Trout baked in the oven, serve immediately after baking.

Bon Appetite!

HEALTHY SALADS & SEAFOOD

Salad with avocado, pineapple, and onions

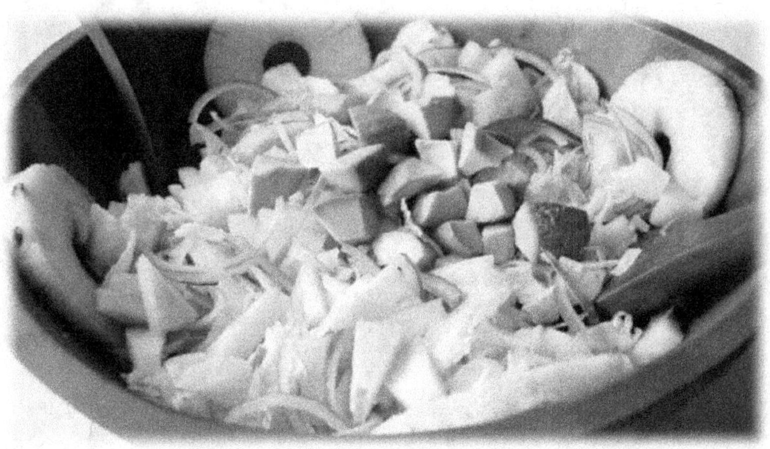

Ingredients (4 servings):

- 1 avocado
- 1 onion
- 6 slices of pineapple
- 1 lemon

Cooking instruction:

In the first instance, you should chop the onion rings. Then the avocado should be cut into small cubes. Now, you can add the lemon juice and mix thoroughly. After that, chop the pineapple into small pieces. Then, you should fry it in sunflower oil until they become golden. Next, you should cool the fried pineapple down. Then place the avocado, pineapple, onion in a bowl and add a little olive oil and the lemon juice. Mix thoroughly. Add the pepper to taste. Well done! Serve immediately.

Bon Appetite!

Salad with scallops and tomatoes

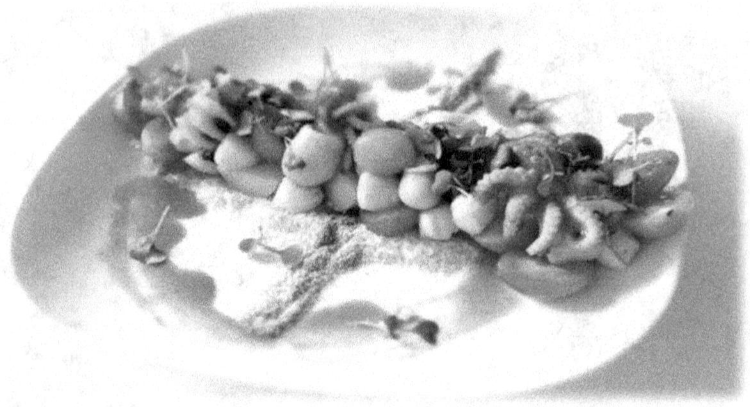

Ingredients (8 servings):

- 100 g of scallops
- 2 tomatoes
- 1 onion red
- half a lemon
- 1.5 teaspoon of mustard in beans
- 0.5 teaspoon of olive oil
- pepper to taste
- greens to taste

Cooking instruction

In the first instance, you should defrost the scallops in a deep container. After that, cut half a lemon into slices and remove the stones from the lemon pulp. Then gently lay the lemon in a bowl and crumble all the ingredients so that the seafood is soaked with lemon juice. Of course, you can use lemon juice, but then the seafood will not permeate with the scent of the peel. Then add black pepper. Mix again and leave for 15-20 minutes. At this time, you should wash the tomatoes, and cut out the green core. After that, cut tomatoes in circles and put on a plate. Peel the red onions from the peel, then rinse and cut in half. You should use only half of the vegetable. Cut it in half rings and lay them on the tomato layer. Then spread on a layer of onion marinated scallops. After that, you should slice the lemon slices into small pieces and layout on the dish. Do not forget to decorate the salad with fresh herbs, for example, dill, Rocca salad, basil or parsley. Add a little salt. In addition, add mustard and vegetable oil. Olive oil is more suitable for this salad. Well done!

Bon Appetite!

Shrimp with spinach

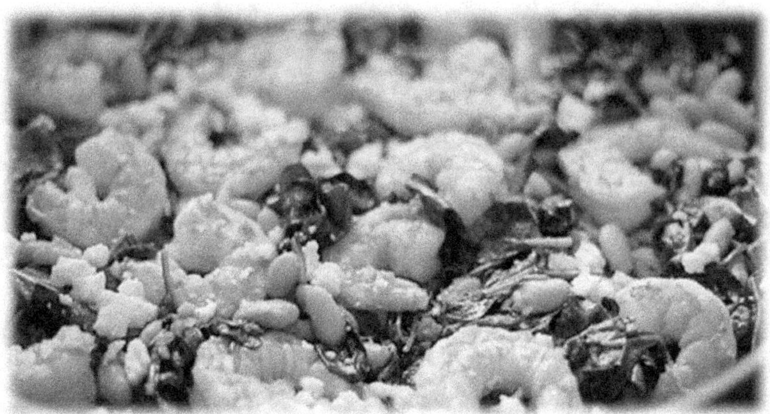

Ingredients (8 servings):

- spinach
- onion
- sage
- butter
- black pepper
- shrimp
- garlic
- olive oil

Cooking instruction:

In the first instance, you should chop onion, sage, and garlic. Next, you need to warm up the frying pan and add a piece of butter and a little olive. This mixture is very tasty and more useful. In addition, the butter does not burn. Add the chopped onion to the melted butter and fry it a little. After the onion is fully fried, you should add spinach. Then add pepper to taste. All ingredients should be cooked for no more than 2-3 minutes. Then transfer the stewed vegetables to a separate bowl. In the same frying pan, you should throw a piece of butter, a little olive, and sage with garlic. After the garlic gives a smell, add the shrimps to the frying pan. If shrimp raw they should be cooked for 3-5 minutes until cooked. Then turn off the fire. Cover the frying pan with a lid and leave the shrimp for a few minutes to soak up the smells. Well done!

Bon Appetite!

Salad with mussels and pine nuts

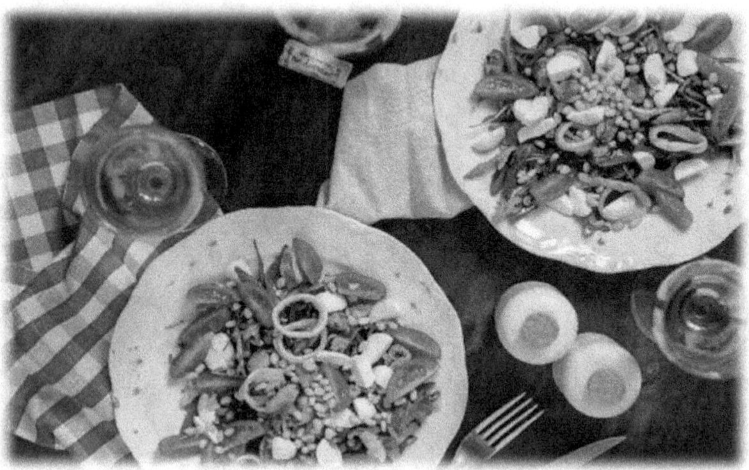

Ingredients (9 servings):

- 100 g of frozen mussels
- 50 g of frozen squid rings
- 100 g of Rocca salad
- 8 pieces of cherry tomatoes
- 50 g of pine nuts
- 10 g of Provençal herbs
- 10 ml of olive oil
- 10 ml of soy sauce
- black pepper to taste

Cooking instruction

In a preheated frying pan fry the mussels and squid rings. Then you should cut the tomatoes into quarters. Mix in a separate bowl of olive oil, soy sauce, and Provencal herbs. You can make a mixture of herbs by yourself, for example, mix basil, rosemary, marjoram and other herbs that you like. Rocca salad can be crushed by hand, or you can leave the leaves whole. Mix all the ingredients and sprinkle with pine nuts. Well done! Serve immediately.

Bon Appetite!

Baked lobster with herbs

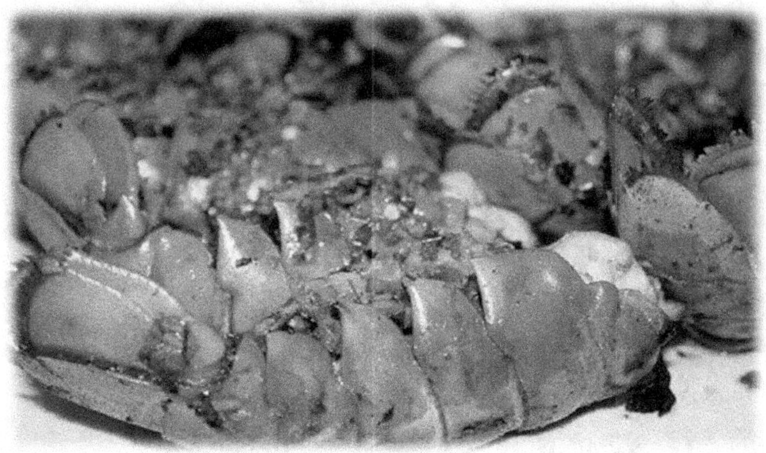

Ingredients (9 servings):

- 500 g of lobsters
- 1-2 cloves garlic
- 2 tablespoons of olive oil
- black pepper to taste
- a few twigs of coriander
- a few twigs of parsley
- a few twigs of rosemary
- 1 tablespoon of lemon juice
- slices of lemon as desired

Cooking instruction

In the first instance, you should finely chop the fresh herbs. After that put the chopped herbs into a deep bowl. Then you should crush the garlic and add it to the bowl. In addition, you should add olive oil and lemon juice. Add pepper to taste. Stir all the ingredients thoroughly until a homogeneous mass appears. Put the lobsters into a dish. You should grease them with the sauce. Then leave the lobsters to marinate for a while, from time to time continue to grease by the sauce. Place the foil on the baking tray and lay out the lobsters. Now you should grease them with sauce again. Bake in preheated to 220°C oven for 10 minutes. After 5 minutes, you should turn over lobsters add the sauce on the other side. Well done! Serve immediately.

Bon Appetite!

Chicken Breast with Persimmon

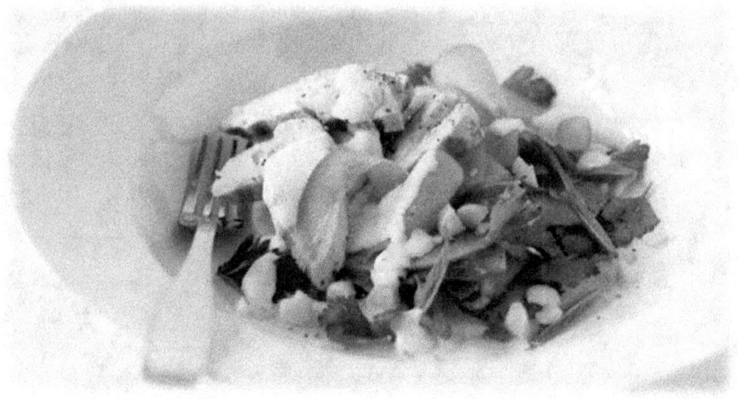

Ingredients (9 servings):

- 500 g of chicken breast
- 100 g of boiled white mushrooms
- 1 persimmon
- 1 onions
- 1 teaspoon of walnuts
- 150 ml of low-fat cream
- spices for chicken
- fresh herbs to taste
- vegetable oil

Cooking instruction:

In the first instance, you should chop the chicken meat into medium-sized pieces. Put the sliced meat in a bowl. Then slice onions into rings and add to the chopped meat. After that, add the spices for the chicken. Stir well. Now, you should place the bowl in the refrigerator for one hour. In one hour, heat a frying pan. Next, fry the meat with onions until the chicken turns white. Then add hot water, and simmer the meat on a low heat under the closed lid for 15 minutes. After that, chop boiled white mushrooms. A persimmon should be cut into large cubes. Well done! Now, grind the walnuts and put all the ingredients in the frying pan. Mix thoroughly. Then pour the low-fat cream into the frying pan and simmer the dish on a low heat for 15 minutes. Finally, you can decorate the dish with fresh herbs to taste. Serve immediately.

Bon Appetite!

Chinese Pak Choy cabbage with Shrimps

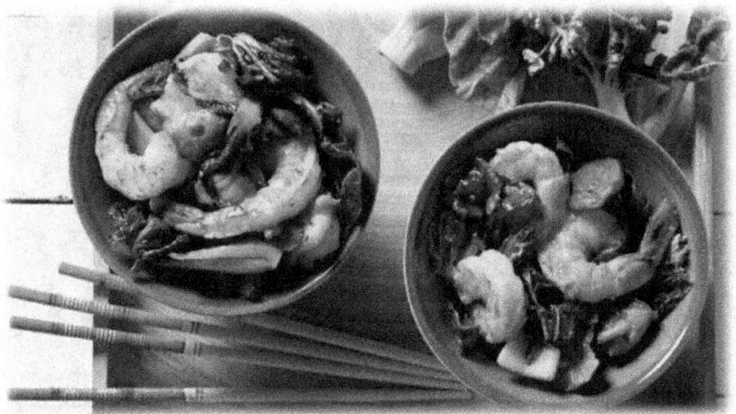

Ingredients (7 servings):

- 1 Chinese Pak Choy cabbage
- 70 g of shrimps without shells
- 1 tablespoon of vegetable oil
- 1 tablespoon of soy sauce
- 1/2 teaspoon of sesame
- 1 tablespoon of sake
- 200 ml of water for thawing shrimps

Cooking instruction

In the first instance, you should boil the water in a saucepan and place the shrimp. After that, add seafood bring water to a boil. Then turn off the heat and leave the seafood to cool in the water for 5 minutes. Next, you should clean Pak Choy cabbage. After that, remove the leaves from the stem and cut out the core. Now, you can fry sesame in oil on a high heat. After that, put shrimps and Pak Choy cabbage into a frying pan. Then, you should add soy sauce and sake. Fry over high heat with intensive stirring for several minutes. Well done! Serve immediately!

Bon Appetite!

Salad with fresh vegetables

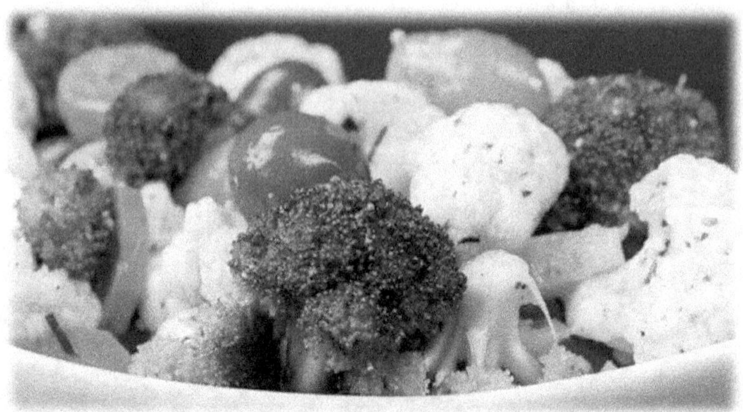

Ingredients (8 servings):

- 350 fresh broccoli
- 2 fresh tomatoes
- 2 fresh cucumbers
- 1 fresh Bulgarian pepper
- 3 tablespoons of olive oil
- juice of half a lemon
- pepper to taste
- 1-2 cloves of garlic

Cooking instruction

In the first instance, you should use only fresh vegetables. Slice tomatoes, cucumbers and bell peppers into cubes. Then break the fresh broccoli into small pieces, and cut the thick stems into circles. The core you should cut and discard. After this place all the chopped vegetables in a large salad bowl, and add the olive oil and juice of half a lemon. Then add the salt to taste and mix well the chopped vegetables. Crush the garlic and add to all the ingredients in the bowl. In addition, you can add the powdered pepper to taste. Thoroughly stir. Well done! Serve immediately!

Bon Appetite!

Salad with shrimps, quail eggs, and black olives

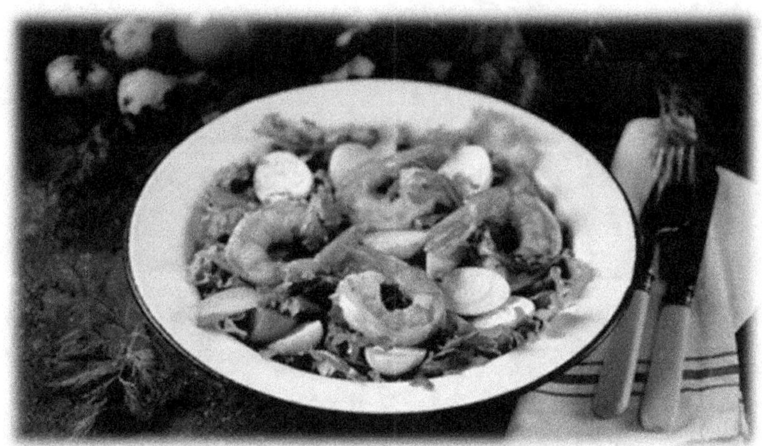

Ingredients (11 servings):

- 300 g of shrimps
- 150 g of black olives
- 1 lemon
- 1 onion
- 3 soup spoons of vinegar
- 5 quail eggs
- 50 g of herbs
- 100 g of lettuce
- 3 soup spoons of olive oil
- 5 cherry tomatoes
- pepper to taste

Cooking instruction

In the first instance, you should marinate the chopped onion in vinegar for 20-30 minutes. Then boil the water in a saucepan and throw in boiling water fresh shrimps. Net pour a little lemon juice. In 1 minute after boiling, remove the saucepan from the heat. Then boil the quail eggs. You should cook quail eggs for 3 minutes after boiling. After that, cool the eggs under cold water and then clean them from the shell. Now you can place the ingredients in a bowl and add the chopped black olives, cherry tomatoes, and leaves of fresh lettuce. After that, add olive oil and lemon juice. In addition, you can decorate the shrimps with lemon slices, herbs, quail eggs and pepper to taste. Well done! Serve immediately!

Bon Appetite!

HEALTHY DINNERS

Cherry dumplings

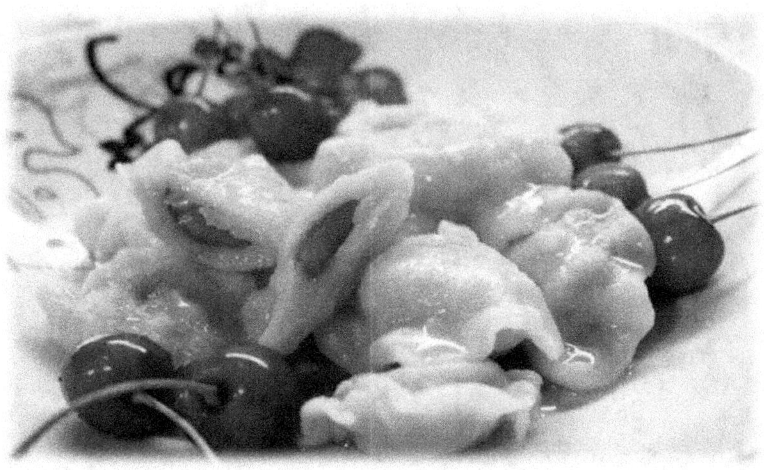

Ingredients (6 servings):

For the dough:
- 3 cups flour
- 1 glass of water
- 2-3 tablespoons of vegetable oil

For filling:
- 500 g of cherry
- 100 g of sugar
- 2-3 tablespoons of flour

Cooking instruction:

In the first instance, you should remove the stones from the cherry, and mix with sugar and flour. After that, mix the flour with warm water, salt and vegetable oil. Then knead the dough for dumplings. Place the dough in a plastic bag and leave for an hour. Thinly roll the dough. The thickness should be about 2 mm. Then cut the dough into small squares. In the middle of each square, put the cherry and pat the edges of the dough. Then bring the water to a boil. You should salt water slightly. After, place the dumplings in a pan and cook until they rise from the bottom of the pan. Well done! Serve immediately!

Bon Appetite!

Risotto with shrimps

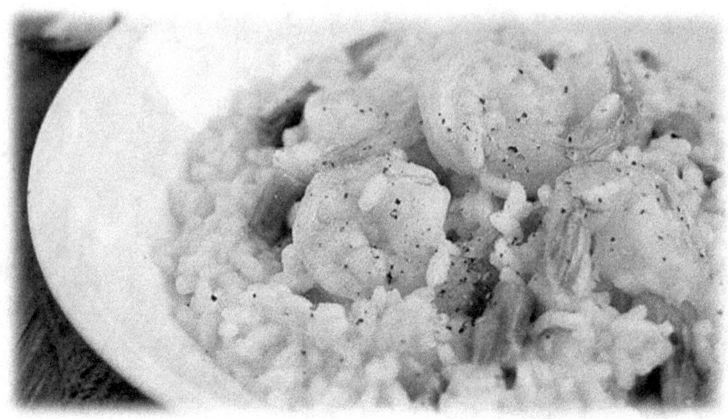

Ingredients (5 servings):

- 1 cup of rice
- 100 – 150 ml of cream (no fat)
- 150 g of shrimp
- 200 g of white mushrooms
- 3 cloves of garlic

Cooking instruction:

In the first instance, you should cook the rice for 20 minutes. After this, chop the white mushrooms and fry them for 2 minutes on a low heat. Add the shrimp to the white mushrooms and fry for 2 minutes on a low heat. Fill a little cream. Salt and pepper you should add to taste. After this, simmer the shrimps with vegetables. Then add the garlic to the shrimp. Wait until the cream soaks into the contents. Add the cooked rice and a little cream to the shrimps, and fry for another 2-3 minutes. Then place all the ingredients in the pan and cook for 25 minutes. Well done! Now, you can enjoy a delicious dinner.

Bon Appetite!

Chicken breast with mushrooms

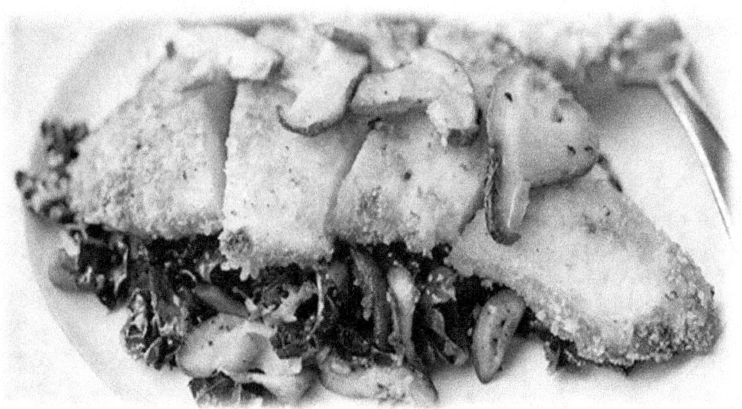

Ingredients (8 servings):

- 500 g of chicken breast
- 100 g of boiled mushrooms
- 1 onion
- 1 teaspoon of walnuts
- chicken spices
- vegetable oil
- fresh herbs
- pepper to taste

Cooking instruction

In the first instance, you should chop the chicken breast into small pieces. Then chop an onion into rings and add to the pieces of chicken. After that, add the chicken spices and salt. Stir thoroughly and place a bowl of meat in the refrigerator not less than for 50 minutes. At the same time add the vegetable oil into a pan, and fry the meat with onions until the chicken pieces become white color. Then add 30 ml of water. You should simmer the meat on a low heat for 20 minutes. After that, you should chop boiled mushrooms and grind walnuts. Then add all the ingredients to the pan. You should simmer the chicken breast and mushrooms on a low heat about for 7-15 minutes. At the end of cooking, do not forget salt and fresh herbs to taste. Well done! Serve immediately.
Bon Appetite!

Turkey steaks

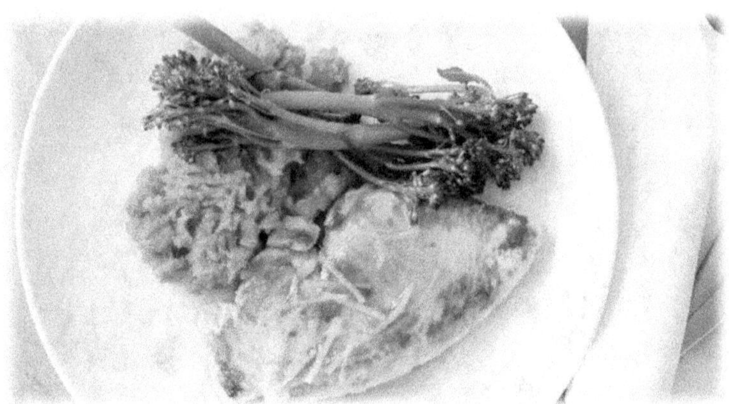

Ingredients (4 servings):

- 500 g of turkey fillet
- 1 teaspoon of black pepper
- sprigs of parsley
- vegetable oil

Cooking instruction:

In the first instance, you should cut the turkey fillet into steaks not more than one cm. After that, you should add salt and pepper to taste. Oil the baking dish with vegetable oil and put the turkey steaks on it. After that, you should preheat the oven. Place the baking dish with the turkey steaks in the oven. You should bake the meat in the oven at 220 ° C for 15 minutes. Well done! After baking, do not forget to decorate the turkey steaks with parsley sprigs or any fresh herbs you want. Well done! Serve immediately.

Bon Appetite!

Vegetable stew with mushrooms

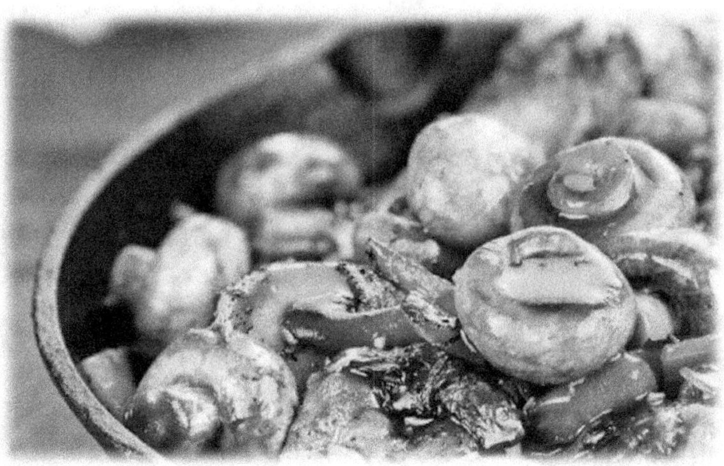

Ingredients (9 servings):

- 2 large sweet peppers of different colors
- 250 g of champignons
- 200 g of asparagus
- 1 onion
- 1-2 cloves of garlic
- a mixture of spices, for example, paprika, ground coriander, basil, marjoram, dill, parsley
- 3 tablespoons soy sauce
- vegetable oil
- fresh herbs

Cooking instruction:

In the first instance, you should place the asparagus in boiling salted water and cook for 7 minutes. Then pour out the boiling water, and pour the asparagus with cold water. After that, you should cut onions and mushrooms. Heat the vegetable oil and fry the onions in a frying pan until a light golden color appears. Add the mushrooms and fry along with the onion until the liquid evaporates. Cut the sweet pepper into strips and add to the mushrooms. Then add salt to taste. In addition, stir well, add spices and crushed garlic. Fry all the ingredients for 5 minutes. Then put the asparagus in a frying pan. You should add soy sauce and mix thoroughly. Then cover the frying pan with a lid and cook over low heat for 2-3 minutes. Well done! Do not forget to decorate the dish with fresh herbs.

Bon Appetite!

Fried rice with vegetables

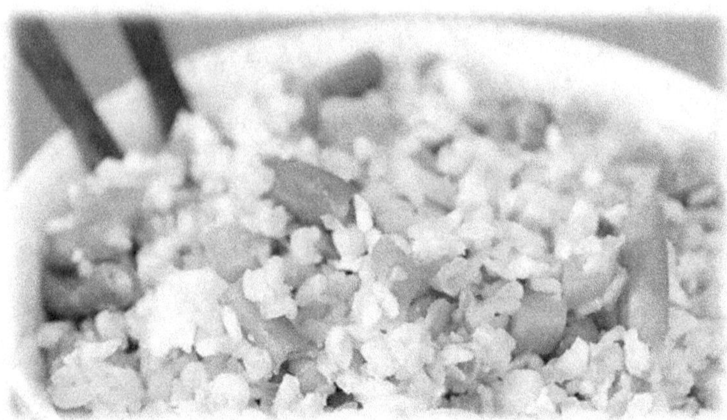

Ingredients (8 servings):

- 4 cups of cooked rice
- 150 g of corn
- 150 g of peas
- 3 eggs
- 2 tablespoons of sesame oil
- 2 cloves of garlic
- 1 tablespoon of ginger
- fresh herbs to taste

Cooking instruction:

In the first instance, you should heat one tablespoon of sesame oil over medium heat. Fry chopped garlic and ginger for one minute. Then add the eggs and mix thoroughly. You should fry them for 1-2 minutes. Add the rice, one tablespoon of sesame oil and reduce heat. Simmer for a few minutes so that the eggs are combined with rice. Add corn and green peas and fry for another two minutes. Well done! Do not forget to add the fresh herbs to taste.
Bon Appetite!

Baked pork with rosemary

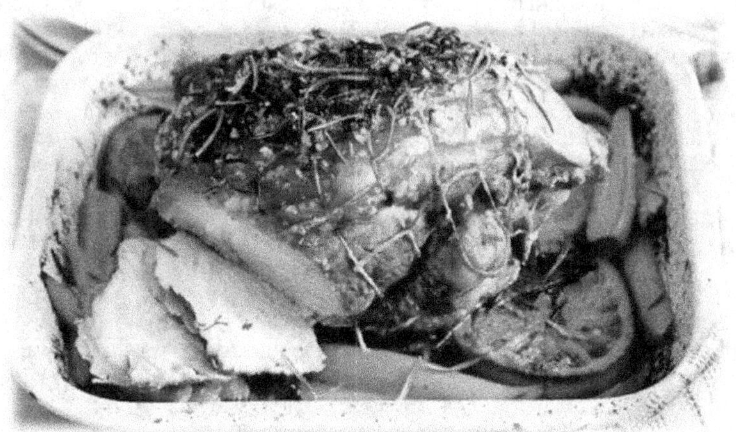

Ingredients (6 servings):

- 1 kg of pork meat
- 1 head of garlic
- 2 tablespoons of olive oil
- 2 tablespoons of dried marjoram
- fresh rosemary
- spices to taste: coriander, oregano, basil, paprika, turmeric, dried garlic, thyme

Cooking instruction:

In the first instance, you should preheat the oven to 200 °C. Then mix 2 tablespoons of olive oil with spices to your taste. Add marjoram and finely chopped rosemary leaves. Oil the meat with oil and spices from all sides. Put the meat in the refrigerator for an hour, then get it out of the refrigerator and warm it to room temperature. Put the meat in a heat-resistant form and pour in 50 ml of water. Next put the head of garlic cut in half. Bake for about 30 minutes. Then turn the meat over and bake for another 30 minutes. If necessary, add water. Remove the meat from the oven and leave it for 10 minutes. Well done!

Bon Appetite!

Conclusion

There is a huge amount of information about healthy nutrition, and it was very difficult to create an overall picture of a balanced diet. Therefore, I made for you a special selection of recipes that will improve your mood, get rid of diseases, increase your overall activity and prolong your life. You should know that my book is your chance to lose weight fast!

Today, I suggest you DASH diet, which allows you to lose weight successfully! In addition, I will teach healthy you cooking philosophy, which could help you reduces weight easy. Sometimes, for quick weight loss, it is very important to change eating habits, although this is not an easy way to success, with my book, it is possible!

In addition, balanced DASH diet can get rid of many diseases or prevent them. You will be able to stabilize your weight effortlessly and restore physical and mental energy. As a result, you will be stronger, and your condition will promote excellent health and beautiful appearance. Therefore, you should try the DASH nutrition system. Who knows perhaps and your way of life will radically change to the best for you!

I am sure that my book will be useful for you. Doubtless, you will find for yourself many useful and tasty healthy dishes on the pages of this book. I wish you with pleasure to pass the way to ideal health, optimal weight, and inexhaustible vital energy.

You should read my book, and make your life easy and happy.

Good luck!

Author's Afterthoughts

Thanks ever so much to each of my cherished readers for investing the time read this book!

I know you could have picked from many other books but you chose this one. So big thanks for downloading this book and reading all way to the end.

If you enjoyed this book or received value from it, I'd like to ask you for a favor. Please take a few minutes to post an honest and heartfelt review on Amazon.com Your support does make a difference and to benefit other people.